Hypothyroidism and Essential Oils:

How Aromatherapy can help regulate hypothyroidism and other tips

Table of Contents

It's your thyroid...

Those words hit you like a punch in the gut. You never expected to have hypothyroidism. You were hoping it was something else, but as your doctor was explaining it to you and writing the prescriptions you would need, you began to wonder if there was anything in the natural health field that could help you. You started looking online for advice, but the amount and contradicting information has your head spinning. There are sites that say herbs and essential oils work, and other sites say that it's pseudoscience and there is not possible way that taking the natural health way will work.

This book is formatted to give you all the information you've been looking for when it comes to taking care of yourself and your thyroid by including essential oils and medical information to back it up. So, if you are ready to take control of your health and your thyroid, you need this book.

You're on your way...

You've purchased a book that will put you on the path to learning more about your thyroid and how to manage hypothyroidism. Take note I am not a licensed Naturopath. The information I gathered for this book comes from years of self-study and reading studies and findings from experts on the subject. By purchasing this book, I hope you have already been to a licensed physician and have been diagnosed with the condition. If not, please, do so. Self diagnosing can be dangerous and lead to more health problems down the road. This book will:

• Explain the function of a thyroid.

• Explain what hypothyroidism is.

• List Essential oils that can help the body regulate thyroid function.

• Provide Aromatherapy recipes you can use to help treat your condition.

• Provide dietary advice on what foods you can add to your diet to help you feel better.

Chapter 1 - Your Thyroid

It doesn't look like much, but it is one of the most important glands in the endocrine system. It takes the trace amounts of iodine you intake naturally through food and turns it into two hormones which control metabolism, but that isn't the only thing it does. Those hormones it produces also helps with regulating functions like:

-Inhaling and exhaling
-Your heart rate
-Part of your nervous system
-Weight gain and loss
-Muscle fortitude
-Monthly women's cycles
-Your temperature
-HDL and LDL levels, and
-a ton more.

You can begin to see how taking care of your thyroid can keep you feeling and being at your best. Your thyroid communicates with your pituitary and hypothalamus glands to regulate those hormones. If something happens to the communication, your thyroid can produce less of the hormones, T3 (triiodothyronine) and T4 (thyroxine), which leads to hypothyroidism.

You're trip to the doctor to find out what was going on was because you were experiencing one or more of the following signs:

-You've been having problems sleeping.

-You're constantly tired, feeling like you've been up for days.

-Your skin is very dry and so is your hair.

-You're depressed when you did not used to be.

-You're more intolerant to the cold than you used to be.

-If you're a woman, you've noticed your periods are uncharacteristically heavy.

-You're having a lot of pain in your muscles and joints.

These are all signs of hypothyroidism.

If you haven't been to the doctor, you need to schedule thyroid function tests to be sure that it is your thyroid that is not acting right. Self diagnosis is not recommended as many of the symptoms above can also be related to other illnesses as well. It is always better to be safe than sorry, and if you feel you need a second opinion, then get one. It is your health, and that is nothing to play guessing games with.

Chapter 2 – Aromatherapy

One cannot talk about essential oils without talking about Aromatherapy. Aromatherapy has been around for many millennia. In fact, it dates back to Ancient Egypt. It was rediscovered when a French chemist, having burned his arm severely, dipped his arm in a vat of lavender essential oil and the arm came out with little to no burn marks or scarring. From there, an old holistic practice was born again. There some things you will need to know before we continue:

-Do not take them internally. Essential oils are the most concentrated form of the plant and are highly toxic when ingested without adding them to recipes.

-Do not use them undiluted. There are some companies that would have you believe you can use them without diluting them with something because of their strength or grade. This is simply not true. You can develop contact dermatitis if you use essential oils in this manner.

-Always look for the Latin name of the essential oil. One common name for something can refer to many different types of plants, and that is why I include the Latin name of the essential oils in this book.

-Though some will say you can stop taking your prescribed medications, I do not. I do recommend you write down how your body feels and how the symptoms become better or worse as you try different essential oils. Everybody is different and thus will react differently to the oils and blends.

-Essential oils are not a cure-all. This is not a book that will tell you essential oils are a magic pill of sorts that will miraculously take care of your hypothyroidism.

It is for this reason some of the oils may not directly treat the condition, but provide relief for some of the symptoms.

Essentials oils need to be diluted with carrier, or base, oils, in order to be used topically. Here are a few you can find in health food stores that are affordable:

- Sweet Almond Oil is the most widely used oil on the market. It is loaded with omega fatty acids and vitamins.

- Apricot Kernel Oil is the second most used oil. This is partly because it is interchangeable with Sweet Almond and many people Apricot if they have nut allergies.

-Olive oil is another one you can use, but it is better to dilute it with one of the oils above.

In a pinch, you can use vegetable oil, but it is better to use one of the three above.

The Essential Oils

Cedarwood, Atlas (Cedrus atlantica)

In blends with other essential oils, it can help balance hormones and is recommended to combat the fatigue that comes with the condition. It aids in relieving stress. Do not use while pregnant.

Clary Sage (Salvia sclarea)

This is a good essential oil for balancing the hormones. It also helps with fatigue and concentration problems and memory. Use in small doses and sparingly.

Frankincense (Boswellia carterii)

Adding this oil to blends will help with depression, and mental fatigue.

Geranium (Pelargonium graveolens)

This is another essential oil that helps with hormone balancing and moods. It also helps with stress, depression, and anxiety attacks.

Jasmine (Jasminum grandiflorum officinale)

This is another good essential oil for evening out moods and mood swings and helping with fatigue, anxiety and depression.

Lemongrass (Cymbopogon citratus)

This essential oil is good for detoxing the thyroid and helps to combat physical and mental fatigue.

Myrrh (Commiphora myrrha)

This oil calms the nerves and helps to reduce the inflammation that happens with the condition.

Myrtle (Myrtus communis)

This essential oil is famous for helping regulate hormones in the body. It helps to stabilize emotions and moods as well as exhaustion, both mental and physical.

Peppermint (mentha piperita)

This helps with apathy, exhaustion, and inflammation of thyroid. It also helps to maintain concentration and mental acuity.

Rosemary (Rosmarinus officinalis)

This oil also has a balancing effect on the hormones. It helps to detoxify the system, maintain mental acuity, and also helps to improve memory. It also used to help in cases of high stress to calm the nervous system. It should not be used with people that are hypertensive and not by pregnant women.

Spearmint (mentha spicata)

This is good in cases of nervous tension, migraines, and fatigue. It helps to calm the nerves.

Ylang Ylang (cananga odorata)

This oil targets anxiety and stress in the system to help with the condition. It is mainly used as a sedative, but also helps with depression and physical exhaustion.

Reflexology Points

Reflexology has been around as long as acupuncture. By applying diluted oils and blends to the points for the thyroid, thymus, and pituitary glands, you can help affect the thyroid in a positive way. Use small circles to massage the blend into the points, and then put on socks to keep the oils on the skin longer. It is best to do this before bed.

Chapter 3 - The Preparations and Blends

Now that we have the information out of the way, let's get into how to make the blends you will be using and how much of the essential oils you can use in each blend.

Notes: Essential oils, or how long they last, is measured in notes: Top, Middle, and Base notes. Here is a breakdown of them.

Top Notes

These are essential oils with a light fragrance and tend to evaporate rapidly. They also have virus fighting properties. In a blend, you would them in concentrations of 15-25%. These are:

-Clary Sage (also a Middle note)
-Lemongrass (also a Middle note)
-Peppermint
-Spearmint

Middle Notes

These essential oils have a balancing effect and their fragrance isn't normally detected immediately in blends. They are used in concentrations of 30-40%. They are:

-Myrtle
-Geranium

Base Notes

These are normally heavy oils and can be readily spotted in blends because of their strong fragrance. They last the longest in the blend and tend to anchor the top notes, helping them to last longer as well. Base notes are used in the largest concentrations, with some exceptions, being 45-55%. These essential oils are:

-Cedarwood
-Clove (not to be used in concentrations more than 5%)
-Frankincense
-Myrrh
-Rosemary
-Ylang Ylang

Tools of the Trade

In all hobbies and interests you will need some basic tools to get started. Luckily, you may already have most, if not, the entire list below in your kitchen.

Glass Mixing Bowls

These are keys in mixing up your blends for some of the preparations. Glass is best because there are no metallic properties the essential oils or carrier oils can leech from the bowl that may change the composition of the blend being made.

Measuring cups and spoons

These are mainly to measure the essential and carrier oils.

Food Scale

You will run across dry ingredients that will need to be measured precisely. A food scale is great for this purpose.

Glass containers with lids

These are to store your blends that you can make in large quantities to keep on hand.

Labels

This is to make sure you know what you have put in the containers so you know when you use them.

Glass Double Boiler

For a couple of the preparations, you will need to use a Bain Marie method to melt ingredients. If you do not have a double boiler that is made of glass, you can place a heavy duty glass bowl in a stock pot and add water around it for the Bain Marie.

Sifter

This will come in handy when making preparations with dry ingredients that tend to clump. If you do not have a sister, you can use a course strainer to the same effect.

Whisk or mixing spoon

You will have to mix your dry ingredients with the liquid ones evenly. To do this, you will need either a whisk or spoon. I would recommend a wooden spoon, if you prefer to use spoons as they do not have glass or plastic whisks.

Diffuser or Candle Warmer

Diffusers are used to disperse the essential oil blends into the air. If you do not have one or can't afford one, using a candle warmer or potpourri warmer will do the trick.

The Preparations

There are many ways to mix and prepare essential oils. From lip balms, to facial masks, you can easily incorporate them into over 20 different products, but we've narrowed the list down a bit for the purposes of this book.

Bath and Mineral Salts

Mixture I
1-2 Cups of Epsom Salts or Magnesium Flakes
1/2 Sea Salt
15-20 Drops of an essential oil or EO blend.

Mixture II
1 Cup of Epsom Salts or Magnesium Flakes
1/2 Cup Baking Soda
1/2 Cup Borax
1/2 Cup Sea Salt
15-20 Drops of an essential oil or EO blend.

Massage oil/Roll-on

4 ounce plastic bottle
4 ounces of carrier oil or blend
40-50 Drops of an essential oil or EO blend

Mix all together and place in the bottle. If you are using a roll-on for easier application, just mix and put the remainder in the larger bottle and refill when needed.

Ointments

9 ounces of Petroleum, or non-petroleum jelly (You can find that online)
40-50 Drops of an Essential oil or EO blend

- In a double boiler, melt the jelly in the double boiler.
- Take the glass bowl of the heat and while it is still warm, add the essential oils.
- Place in a container with a tight lid.

Salve

1/2 Cup carrier oil
1 tbsp
2 tbsp shea butter
30 drops of essential oil or EO blend

1. In a double boiler, melt the beeswax and shea butter.
2. Add the oil.
3. Mix well.
4. Wait until it cools to add the essential oils.
5. Place the salve in containers and make sure they are cool before tightening the lid.

Chapter 4 - Adjusting Your Diet

You can't talk about whole-body health without touching on foods that help to feed the thyroid and aid in boosting your thyroids activity.

Fish

Adding more fish to your diet can help benefit your thyroid, not only due to the fatty acids found in fish like wild salmon, trout and tuna, but it also has selenium. Selenium is in high concentrations in your thyroid.

Nuts

These are another food that is high in selenium. They are also easy to portion out and take with you, if you have a busy schedule.

Whole Grains

These can help you regular in your bowel movements, which in turn can help with thyroid help. Steel cut oats, barley, whole wheat are just three of the many options out there. Just talk to your doctor first if you are taking synthetic hormones.

Fresh Fruits and Vegetables

Eating 5-7 servings of these a day are very beneficial to your overall health, as many know, but you will want to limit your intake of vegetables like broccoli and cabbage can reduce your thyroid's ability to process iodine.

Kelp

Otherwise known as seaweed, kelp is rich in iodine, fiber, calcium, and vitamins A, B, C, E, and K. Check with your doctor about the amount of iodine that is safe to intake in your diet as too much can make matters worse.

Dairy

Milk and cheese can help keep up calcium and vitamin D levels.

Beans

High in fiber, antioxidants, complex carbs and vitamins and minerals, beans are also wonderful in helping maintain high energy level to counteract the fatigue many experience with hypothyroidism.

Foods to Avoid

Soy-heavy foods

Though the jury is out on the effect of is flavone in soy, some in the research field say too much soy can make you more susceptible to hypothyroidism. It might impede your ability to assimilate your thyroid medication.

Gluten

This is referring to added gluten in foods and not in whole grains, but it's always good to get tested for gluten intolerance.

Fried Foods/high fat foods

Foods that are fried or food high in saturated fat can make it hard for your body to absorb your medications. They may even impede the production of hormones from your thyroid.

Sweets

Because your metabolism slows down when your thyroid under-produces, you will be more likely to gain weight if you don't watch your intake of sugary foods.

Processed foods

Processed foods are convenient, but they can be high in sodium, which is not good for the thyroid or your blood pressure. There are a lot of websites out there that can help make healthy, and delicious, meals which are quick to make a package.

Hold off on the coffee

Wait for that first cup until about 30 minutes after you've had your medication. The caffeine in the coffee can block your body from absorbing your medicine.

No Alcohol

Alcoholic drinks can throw your thyroid levels off and, in some cases; it can also make it hard on your thyroid to produce its main hormone.

If you still want to drink, every once in a while and in moderation is recommended.

Since all of our bodies are different, I would also suggest keeping a food diary, listing the foods that make you feel good as well as the ones that make you feel worse. This can be the best guide of all.

Chapter 5 - Aromatherapy Recipes

Now, we get into the fun stuff. Here are some recipes you can try at home to help you. Don't stop with these, however. Try some of your own blends. Go online to communities and ask for more advice and more recipes.

Diffuser Recipes

Anxiety and Stress I
5 Drops Atlas Cedarwood EO
3 Drops Geranium EO
2 Drops Myrtle EO

Anxiety and Stress II
5 Drops Jasmine EO
3 Drops Peppermint EO
3 Drops Clary Sage EO

Hormone Balance I
5 Drops Rosemary EO
3 Drops Geranium EO
2 Drops Clary Sage EO

Hormone Balance II
6 Drops Frankincense EO
3 Drops Myrtle EO
1 Drop Clary Sage EO

Fatigue Recipe I
5 Drops Jasmine EO
3 Drops Myrrh EO
2 Drops Lemongrass EO

Fatigue Recipe II

6 Drops Ylang Ylang EO
2 Drops Peppermint EO
2 Drops Lemongrass EO

Bath Salts

Relaxing recipe I
8 Drops Atlas Cedarwood EO
4 Drops Myrrh EO
4 Drops Jasmine EO
4 Drops Geranium EO

Relaxing Recipe II
8 Drops Ylang Ylang EO
6 Drops Myrtle EO
3 Drops Lemongrass EO
3 Drops Clary Sage EO

Invigorating Recipe
8 Drops Frankincense EO
6 Drops Jasmine EO
3 Drops Peppermint EO
3 Drops Spearmint EO

Massage oil

Hormone Oil
4 Ounces of Carrier Oil
15 Drops Myrtle EO
10 Drops Rosemary EO
10 Drops Lemongrass EO
5 Drops Clary Sage EO

Massage in and around the thyroid area and the reflexology points on the feet for the thyroid.

Detox and Anxiety Oil
15 Drops of Ylang Ylang EO
10 Drops of Frankincense EO
10 Drops Geranium EO
10 Drops Jasmine EO
5 Drops Peppermint EO

Ointment

General Purpose I
9 Ounces Unpetroleum Jelly
15 Drops Frankincense EO
15 Drops Atlas Cedarwood EO
10 Drops Myrtle EO
5 Drops Lemongrass EO
5 Drops Clary Sage EO

General Purpose II
9 Ounces Unpetroleum Jelly
15 Drops Ylang Ylang EO
15 Drops Jasmine EO
10 Drops Rosemary EO
5 Drops Peppermint EO
5 Drops Myrrh EO

Chapter 6 - For the Cooks

Here are some quick and easy recipes you can prepare and even package them for taking to work.

Breakfast

Breakfast Smoothie

1/4 C Raw cashews soaked overnight
1/2 Medium Banana
1/2 Medium Red Apple, peeled, cored, and chunked
1/2 C chopped Kale
1/2 Lemon squeezed
1 Cup coconut milk
2 capsules Kelp
Ice
- Strain the water out of the Cashews
- Add the Cashews and the coconut milk to the blender
- Put the blender on liquefy
- Add the fruits
- Add the kale
- Add ice to thicken

Kale and Tomato Omelette

2 Eggs, whipped
2 leaves of kale, cleaned and chopped
1 Roma tomato chopped
1/4 Cup shredded Colby Jack Cheese
1 tsp olive oil
A pinch each of basil, salt, onion powder, rosemary
• Gently heat the Olive oil in the pan
• Add the tomatoes and kale
• Lightly sautee the vegetables
• When warm, pour the whipped eggs and evenly distribute them in the pan.
• Peel back the egg to allow all the of raw egg to cook on one side
• Flip the omelette
• Add the cheese
• Fold over and serve with whole grain or sprouted toast

Banana nut Oatmeal

1 Cup Steel Cut Oats
3 1/2 cups milk
2 medium ripe bananas, the browner spots the better, mashed
1/2 cup chopped walnuts
1 tsp salt
1/2 tsp nutmeg
1 tsp cinnamon
1 tsp vanilla extract
3 tbsp raw honey, or sweeten to taste
• Place the mashed bananas in a pot with the milk.
• Gently heat on medium heat and stir occasionally
• Add the honey, vanilla extract, nutmeg and cinnamon
• Simmer for 10 minutes. Taste the mixture. Add more of the spices to taste.
• Bring the mixture to a slow boil
• Add the oats
• Wait for boil to return, stirring every now and then
• Simmer for 30-40 minutes, until soft.
• Serves 4-6

Lunch

Spinach and Romaine Chicken Salad

1 Handful of washed Baby Spinach
1 handful of chopped Romaine Lettuce
1/2 Cup Red apple, peeled and chopped
1/2 Cup cucumber, peeled and chopped
1 medium Roma tomato chopped
1/4 Cup sliced Almonds
1/4 Cup sliced Strawberries
Onion powder
Garlic powder
Finely ground sea salt
3 ounces boneless, skinless chicken breast
2 tsp Extra Virgin olive oil
2 tbsp raspberry vinaigrette
• Season the chicken breast to taste with the powdered onion, garlic and light salt
• Heat a pan to medium heat and add the Olive Oil
• Cook the chicken completely
• Shred the chicken
• Chill the chicken
• Mix all the fruits and vegetable together.
• Add the chicken and dressing
• Toss until all of the salad is coated with the dressing
To have it on the go, it makes two burrito sized wraps.

Healthy Chicken Salad

6 Ounces of pre-cooked chicken, preferably baked left-overs
1 Medium Red Apple
1/2 Cup chopped walnuts
1/2 Cup sliced green grapes
2 stalks of celery sliced
1/4 plain Yogurt
- Shred the chicken
- Mix in the fruits, veggies and nuts with the chicken
- Stir in the yogurt

Dinner

Citrus Salmon

3 Ounces of Wild-Caught Salmon
1/4 Cup Fresh Orange Juice
1/4 Cup Fresh Lemon Juice
2 tbsp Minced onion
1 minced garlic clove
- Mix the juices and herbs together
- In a container, add the marinade and Salmon
- Marinate the fish for two hours
- Bake at 350 degrees for 4 minutes per 1/2-inch thickness

Honey Carrots

2 Medium Carrots, cleaned and peeled
1 tbsp butter
2 tbsp raw honey
Pinch of salt
Pinch of cinnamon
- Slice the carrots to 1/8 on an inch
- Heat the butter in a saute pan
- Saute the carrots in the butter until half cooked.
- Add the salt and cinnamon
- Saute a little longer, until they are just about cooked.
- Add the honey.
- Stir to coat the slices of carrot
The carrots should still have a light crunch, but not be soggy.

Apple Roasted Pork Chops

1 1/2 tsp Rubbed Sage
1 tsp minced garlic
1 tsp thyme leaves
1/2 tsp ground Allspice
1/2 paprika
1 tbsp brown rice flour
1 tsp sea salt
4-6 1 inch thick center cut pork chops
1/2 apple juice
1 tbsp brown sugar
1 tbsp olive oil
1 medium onion thinly sliced
1 medium red apples peeled and thinly sliced
• Place onions and apples in a gallon sized freezer bag
• Place 1 tbsp brown sugar in the bag with the remaining ingredients, minus the pork.
• Mix all ingredients well
• Add the pork chops and coat them well.
• Marinate for up to four hours
• Place the pork chops and marinade in a lined baking pan.
• Preheat oven to 400 degrees
• bake for 25 minutes
If you want to make some gravy to go on top, this is where the flour and the rest of the brown sugar come into play.
• Pour the liquid into a pan on the stove
• Use medium heat and a whisk
• Whisk in the rest of the brown sugar
• Add the brown rice flour, 1 1/2 tbsp to thicken the gravy.
• Pour on the pork chops.
Don't throw away those apple peels!

Apple Saffron Rice

4 1/2 Cups Water
2 Cups Brown Rice
1 tbsp sea salt
1/4 medium white onion, minced
1 tsp Vanille Extract
1 generous pinch of saffron
1 tbsp olive oil
Peels from the recipe above
- Add everything but the rice to the water
- Bring the water to a boil
- Add the rice
- bring to boil
- turn to low heat and cover
- Simmer for 40 minutes, or until soft, stirring occasionally.

Quick Snacks

Goat Cheese and Fruit

1/2 Cup of either Strawberries or blue berries
1/4 cup of soft Goat Cheese that has been whipped
• Mix the fruit into the cheese
• Spread on crackers

Quick and easy Fruit Salad

• Take your favorite fruits, peel and chop them
• Add vanilla flavored yogurt

Cashew "Cheese"

I know what you're thinking, but this is a great spread on crackers and sandwiches.
1 Cup raw cashews, soaked overnight
2 tbsp nutritional yeast (health food store)
1 tsp fresh lemon juice (more if you like the taste.
1 tsp tarragon
1/2 tsp sea salt
1/2 tsp ground pepper
1/4 purified water
• Soak the cashews overnight and drain them.
• Place them with the juice, herbs, pepper and salt in a food processor
• As the processor runs, add the water until you get the consistency you want. More water means a thinner spread.
You can experiment with different herbs in the recipe for a different taste every time. If you love garlic, start with one clove.

Chapter 7 - Support and Help

Just because you have been diagnosed with hypothyroidism doesn't mean you have to figure out how to manage it alone. There are tons of resources out there you can use to connect with other people to talk to; recipe sites to help with fitting your changes into your diet, and also sites that can help keep you on track. Here are some to help you out.

Recipe Sites

Everyday health

The Healing Gourmet

These are just two of the many out there. Try new recipes at least twice a week. You will be surprised at what you will like just by giving it a taste.

Support Boards/Groups

Looking for a place to vent? Need to find people to get advice from or give a little advice? There are hundreds of support forums online for hypothyroidism. It's a great way to connect with people and make friends.

Conclusion

There are many things you can do to manage your condition. This book was the start on the path on how to take charge of your condition in conjunction with your existing medications. Please, keep in mind I am not a licensed care giver. I am someone who has studied natural health for over twenty years.

I hope this book serves you well in getting you started on your path to feeling better and being healthier. Don't stop with this book, though. Strike out on your own and seek out more knowledge. You only have one life. Make the most of it while you are here.

www.ingramcontent.com/pod-product-compliance
Lightning Source LLC
Chambersburg PA
CBHW070102260726
48658CB00002B/956